KEGEL EXERCISES FOR WOMEN

A WOMAN'S GUIDE TO KEGEL EXERCISES

HOLLY SAYLES

Table of Contents

CHAPTER ONE

A WOMAN'S GUIDE TO KEGEL EXERCISES

Is there a KEGEL workout?

Exercises of the pelvic floor, also known as kegels or kegel exercises, are an excellent method for enhancing and maintaining normal bowel and bladder function. In order to improve or even eliminate bladder leakage, men and women alike can benefit from performing kegels to strengthen their pelvic floor muscles.

Is KEGELS RIGHT FOR YOU?

Many people find that kegel exercises are an excellent way to maintain or improve the health of their pelvic floor, whether they're trying to alleviate the symptoms of urinary incontinence or not. Many symptoms of bladder prolapse, bladder leakage, and urinary urgency can be alleviated by strengthening and toning the pelvic floor. Women and men with weak pelvic floors may benefit from kegel exercises. Exercises for the pelvic floor can help tighten the muscles and restore their natural role in pelvic organ support and stability.

Kegel exercises, on the other hand, aren't for everyone. In some cases, excessive Kegel exercises may actually do more harm than good.

In some cases, the pelvic floor is too active or tense, leading to pelvic floor disorders. Pelvic floor relaxation is difficult to achieve when this occurs. Pelvic floor hyperactivity may result as a result of this.

Having a tense or active pelvic floor is bad for your health. Having a constantly overactive pelvic floor makes it difficult to contract when you need it, not only because the muscle is fatigued but also because it has limited range of movement. The muscle has already been shortened. Due to the ineffectiveness of the muscles in their response to the situation when you sneeze or if you're trying to avoid an accident when you really need to go, you may end up leaking.

In these cases, Kegel exercises are not recommended for strengthening or enhancing tone. Pelvic floor therapists are the only ones who can tell you whether you have a weak or an overactive pelvic floor, so seeing one before beginning any pelvic floor exercise routine is always recommended.

You can learn how to do a Kegel and, more importantly, how to relax your pelvic floor with the help of a physical therapist. A pelvic floor therapist's job description and what to expect at an appointment can be found here.) There are biofeedback tools that allow you to see or feel how well you're squeezing and ensure that you're engaging the correct muscles during these appointments.

CHAPTER TWO

A WOMAN'S GUIDE TO KEGEL EXERCISES IN ITS ENTIRETY

How can you tell if you're doing Kegels correctly? It can be hard to tell at first, just like any other form of exercise. But if you make it a daily habit, it becomes second nature. The following are some pointers for female kegel exercisers:

WHAT MUSCLES ARE NEEDED?

It is possible to halt the flow of urine mid-stream if you can identify the muscles of the lower abdomen. That's the most challenging part of the exercise. Pelvic floor physical therapy (or PFT) is necessary if you're having trouble pinpointing the correct muscles.

In terms of how many times a day I should do them, I'm not sure.

To begin, tighten your pelvic floor muscles for five seconds while performing with an empty bladder. Take a few deep breaths, and then take a five-second break. Make an effort to complete five repetitions on your first attempt. As you become more comfortable with your new routine, try to keep your contractions to 10 seconds at a time and relax for 10 seconds in between. Ten full Kegels are performed during each session.

You can work up to three full Kegel sessions per day as you gain strength.

Focus on both your fast-twitch and slow-twitch muscle fibers during your workouts.

Focused kegel exercises for the pelvic floor are available for two different types of workouts.

The first exercise is called a quick or short contraction, which is a fast twitch muscle exercise. In order to prevent urine leakage, it uses fast-twitch muscle fibers to compress the urethra quickly.

For these exercises, the muscles are tightened for only a few milliseconds before being released. While performing these exercises, be sure to breathe normally.

This exercise, known as a long hold contraction, targets the supporting strength and endurance of slow-twitch muscle fibers.

The muscles you used for the quick contractions will now be gradually tightened, lifted, and held for several seconds in order to perform these contractions.

Holding a contraction for more than a few seconds may be difficult at first. Each long contraction should last 10 seconds, followed by a 10-

second pause to avoid overtaxing the muscles.

WHAT TO BE ON THE LOOKOUT FOR

Take care not to engage your abdominal, thigh, or buttock muscles during this exercise. Holding your breath is also a bad idea. To avoid overstressing the rest of your body, take a deep breath during the exercises. When holding a breath, it may be helpful to count the number of seconds you are holding it out loud.

- **DO YOUR EXERCISES AT LEAST THREE TIMES PER DAY!**

Every day, try to complete at least three sets of ten repetitions per set. Eventually, once you've mastered the technique.

It's important to give yourself a boost of confidence.

Starting out with kegel exercises can be a bit awkward. However, the more time you put into it, the better your muscles will feel and the better your bladder health will be. Additionally, kegels have been shown to enhance sexual pleasure. Yes!

Two or three times a day, do one set of ten short contractions and one set of ten long contractions as an effective kegel workout. Always keep in mind that quantity is secondary to quality. It's better to perform a smaller number of kegels correctly than to perform a large number of kegels in an incorrect manner. Depending on the severity of your condition, you may see results in as little as four weeks or as long as a year.

Increase the weight of the dumbbell you're using for arm curls or other kegel exercises to provide resistance against muscle contractions as a training aid. A doctor's prescription is required for some of these aids, while others can be purchased over the counter.

There are a plethora of options available today, some of which require a vaginal insert while others are as simple as putting on a pair of shorts. Before using any of these gadgets, make an appointment with your physical therapist or doctor.

CHAPTER THREE

TACKLE YOUR
DEVELOPMENT WITH
CARE.

Use our pelvic floor exercise tracker to see how much better you get each week. To keep you motivated, this sheet will also allow you to keep track of how your Kegels and pelvic floor strength improve over the course of a year.

You can also use this tracker to show your insurance company that you've tried Kegel exercises on your own before they'll cover the cost of a Kegel device, which can help you save money.

Signs of an increase in the pelic floor's tensile strength

Signs of an increase in the pelic floor's tensile strength

It takes time to strengthen your pelvic floor. Look for these signs as a sign that your pelvic floor muscle exercises are working and that you are on your way to better bladder health rather than being discouraged if you are not able to control your bladder as quickly as you would like.

More time between visits to the restroom.

• There are fewer "accidents"

Increased endurance and/or volume of contractions

• Comfortable underwear that doesn't feel like it's always wet.

• Getting a good night's rest

Biofeedback therapy may be helpful for women and men who have difficulty performing kegel exercises on their own. Many people can improve their pelvic floor muscle strength, tone, and function with the help of a nurse specialist or pelvic floor therapist and a good regimen.

You must remember that incontinence and pelvic floor symptoms are almost always treatable and should not be considered normal. With these exercises, it does not matter how long you have had your symptoms. It's never too late to try Kegels, no matter how long you've had leaks for. It could be 1 month or 10 years.

Squeeze it into your schedule as often as possible. The majority of the time, doing Kegels will help alleviate your symptoms. Specialists may be able to help if you're not getting the results you want.

Better Sex with Kegel Exercises

In order to improve your sex life, you should practice Kegels.

Because the pelvic floor muscles are critical to arousal, pleasure, and orgasm response, it is important to keep them strong and healthy.

A woman's orgasm response is amplified when her muscles are firm, and this firmness can enhance the pleasure she gets from her partner. Additionally, there are a number of advantages.

Sexual satisfaction can be improved by strengthening the pelvic floor muscles through specific exercise.

Exercises known as Kegels are often performed with Kegel weights, cones, eggs or balls in order to strengthen the pelvic floor muscles.

The time required for each workout is greatly reduced by the use of these devices. Vaginal weight sets are an excellent option for women who are serious about improving their physical appearance in that area. Our Intimate Rose weight system is the best in the business.

Next, we'll go over the fundamentals of the Kegel, and if you're more visual, there are images for each exercise!

THE BASIC STRENGTHENING OF THE PELVIC FLOOR

Basics of Kegel

An effective Kegel is one in which you pull your urethra up and into your body as if it were a telescope. It is important to avoid squeezing your buttocks too tightly or contracting your abdomen too much during this exercise. Additionally, the importance of inhalation and exhalation can't be overstated.

In order to properly contract the muscles, holding your breath will put pressure on the bladder and the pelvic floor, making it difficult. Relaxedly inhale for a few seconds and then exhale like you're blowing out birthday candles while simultaneously performing the Kegel exercise.

To perform a Kegel, get comfortable in a chair or lie down. Relax and inhale. Take a deep breath out, squeeze your glutes for five seconds, and then let go. Do this ten times. Do it four times a day. Work your way up from a 5-second hold to a 10-second hold gradually.

Pelvic floor strength can be improved with more challenging exercises once you have mastered Kegels. While performing a Kegel, these exercises can be performed. The goal is to be able to maintain the Kegel throughout the entire range of motion.

Using Bridge and Kegel

Place your knees bent and feet hip-width apart on the floor. Breathe in through your nose.

As you exhale, perform a Kegel and raise your hips 2-4 inches off the floor. Then lower them back down. Relax your muscles by inhaling and then exhaling.

Perform a full set of ten. Repetition is key here.

Kegel and March together

Place your knees bent and feet hip-width apart on the floor. Breathe in through the nose. Breathe out and do a Kegel while simultaneously lifting your right leg to a 90-degree angle, then slowly lowering it.

Your pelvis should not move. Exhale and do a Kegel on the right leg, then inhale and do the same on the left, going back and forth. Keep in mind that lifting the leg should be a slow and continuous movement, not a pause.

Perform ten reps on each leg separately. Repetition is key here.

CHAPTER FOUR

PROGRESSING WITH THE KEGEL RESISTANCE DEVICE.

Intimate Rose's vaginal exercise weights can be used to increase the difficulty of these Kegel exercises for women. Begin by inserting the white vaginal weight into the vagina as you would a tampon to determine the appropriate weight for exercise. Try to hold your weight in the vagina for a minute while standing up.

For 20 minutes, walk around your house doing chores as you normally would with your clothes on and the weight inserted if this is possible. On a subsequent day, try this with the next heaviest weight, if it's possible.

Using the weight that you were able to tolerate for 20 minutes should be sufficient to perform the Basic Kegel exercise if it slips out of your hands and into your underwear.

Perform these exercises at least three times a week for best results. After a few weeks, you might be ready to go up a weight class.

Sexy KEGEL TRAINING FOR IMPROVED PERFORMANCE

Pelvic floor strength can be improved even further by performing the exercises listed below in an upright, gravity-defying position. The following exercises should be performed three to five times per week, using a vaginal weight that you can hold for 20 minutes.

Kegel in a standing position

Stand tall with good posture, feet hip-width apart, with the weight in.

Relax your muscles by taking a deep breath in. Once you're done inhaling, do a Kegel and hold the Kegel for 5 seconds while exhaling. Take a deep breath and let your muscles relax. Do this ten times.

Performing the Kegel Standing Heel Raise

With your vaginal weight in, use the counter of your kitchen as a support.

Take a deep breath and let your muscles relax. Take a deep breath out, perform a Kegel, and slowly rise up onto the balls of your feet before lowering yourself back to the floor slowly and steadily. Inhale and relax your pelvic floor, then exhale and repeat once your feet are back on the floor.

As you raise your feet to your toes and lower them back down, you should be able to feel the Kegel. Do this ten times.

Squat Kegel

With your vaginal weight in, balance and support yourself at your kitchen counter.

Relax your muscles by taking a deep breath in. Kneel to about 45 degrees while pressing your hips backward as if you were going to sit in a chair while exhaling simultaneously. Maintaining the Kegel, rise to your feet. Keeping a Kegel and a gentle exhale throughout the movement is essential. Inhale and let go as soon as you're back on your feet. Do this ten times.

Intimate Rose's kegel weight system is recommended by doctors. If you want to get a tighter vagina, these exercises will help you get there more quickly.

Let's take a quick look at how these exercises can enhance your sex life before we get started.

Strengthening the Pelvic Floor Muscles has numerous advantages.

For both men and women, strong pelvic floor muscles have been shown to improve sexual intercourse. The muscles of the pelvic floor act as a support system for the reproductive organs.

Vaginal or Kegel weights, also known as Kegel exercises, can be added to your workouts to target these muscles and get better results in less time. Our system includes weights, exercise videos, and more so that you can get better results in less time than with other products.

41

THE END

www.ingramcontent.com/pod-product-compliance
Lightning Source LLC
Chambersburg PA
CBHW050621160726
48003CB00003B/1280